Mathematics and Medicine

How Serious is the Injury?

William Sacco
Wayne Copes
Clifford Sloyer
Robert Stark

JANSON PUBLICATIONS, INC. Providence, Rhode Island

Material based on work supported by the National Science Foundation and produced by the committee on Enrichment Modules, Department of Mathematical Sciences, University of Delaware, and Tri-analytics, Bel Air, Maryland.

94 93 92 91 90 89 88   8 7 6 5 4 3 2

Contents

The authors wish to thank Jane Melville and John Graybeal, who helped to
to produce this monograph.

Preface

Picture yourself in this situation. You are a paramedic or ambulance driver attached to a local fire department or civil defense branch.

You have been alerted to the occurrence of a major disaster in your area. Following a general alarm you are en route to the scene and hear this announcement over the radio:

10:00 A.M.

Thirty minutes ago, the city of San Francisco was nearly leveled by the major earthquake scientists have been predicting for the last few years. The quake measured 7.8 on the Richter Scale, with an epicenter only 10 miles outside the heavily populated city.

An estimate of property damage is about 200 billion dollars. No estimate is yet available for loss of life.

The President has declared the area a Disaster Area, and the Red Cross is mobilizing all of its resources to help. Citizens in the area have been warned to boil all water for consumption because of contamination.

Hospitals in the area that are still able to function are swamped with victims. Those injured who are able to are requested to wait 24 hours before attempting to enter the emergency rooms.

All physicians and other medical personnel in the area are requested to report to the nearest hospital to help with the enormous number of injured victims.

You, and many others like you, will have a vital role in determining the ultimate outcome of this life and death situation. For example, paramedics and ambulance drivers must decide where accident victims should be taken. Going to the nearest hospital is not always the best thing to do. The technical term for this decision is *triage*. Suppose a huge earthquake struck. Which patients should be treated first? What a massive sorting problem this would be! In intensive care units as many as 60 measurements are made on patients many times a day. Simple methods need to be developed to use these data so that a patient's condition may be tracked during treatment. Finally, how well does a given hospital or trauma center care for its patients? Methods must be developed for the evaluation of patient care.

What do the problems of patient triage, sorting, tracking, and evaluation of care have in common? All can be attacked by using indices which measure the severity of patient illness or injury. In what follows we will explore in detail many of the indices you might use in dealing with such a disaster as the earthquake mentioned above. We define indices, describe methods of constructing them, and apply them to medical problems. Real data from trauma patients have been used to create the tables and indices, and the role of the mathematician in developing them will become clear.

Triage decisions are influenced by the extent of an accident victim's injuries or condition. The nearest hospital may well not be equipped to render the level of care the victim needs, and valuable time could be lost by first transporting a patient to the nearest hospital and then making a transfer.

In sorting mass casualties, those patients who have no chance of survival must be identified so that doctors do not spend time on them and thereby lose the chance to save others.

Once a patient is placed in the proper facility for his or her needs, the patient's condition must be tracked carefully. As many as 60 physiological and biochemical measurements may be made on each patient each day. Such information must be readily available to physicians and nurses in a form that is easily read. Such tracking is used as an indicator of how well or poorly therapy is working and dictates whether new therapies should be tried, and when.

Evaluation of patient care is another aspect of medical treatment in which indices are invaluable. Graphic displays can help a hospital assess its quality of care by identifying unexpected deaths or survivals. A hospital can readily compare its performance from year to year, as well as check its performance against that of another hospital which treats patients with similar injury severities.

Expanded definitions of the terms triage, sorting, tracking, and quality of patient care appear in Appendix I.

When you complete this monograph, you will be on the frontier of the research in this exciting application of mathematical science.

Part I
INDICES — DISCUSSION

A. Indices in General

An index is a number, based on one or more measurements, that serves to indicate some sort of condition. For example, a baseball batting average (number of hits/total times at bat) is an index. It is probably the most widely used indicator of the ability of a batter.

1. Name three other indices used to assess the abilities of batters.

   _____

   _____

   _____

2. In many competitions, judges score performance on artistic merit. Name three such competitions.

   _____

   _____

   _____

3. What does a barometer measure? _____

4. What do barometric readings indicate? _____

5. What is the Cost of Living Index? _____

6. What does it indicate? _____

7. What does an oral thermometer measure? _____

8. What does it indicate? _____

All of these quantities are indices. Again, indices are numbers which are indicators of conditions. They are based on one or more measurements.

B. Index Development — An Example

A good index is simple and informative. How is such an index developed? Here is a set of steps which may have led to an index based on body temperature.

- *Observation* — "Hot" head accompanies complaints of sickness.

- *Theory* — Physicians understand theory (infection causes temperature rise) which supports their observation.

- *Measurement Method* — Thermometer invented.

- *Data Collected* — Temperatures taken of healthy and sick persons.

- *Data Analyzed* — Consider the plot of observed temperatures given in Figure 1.

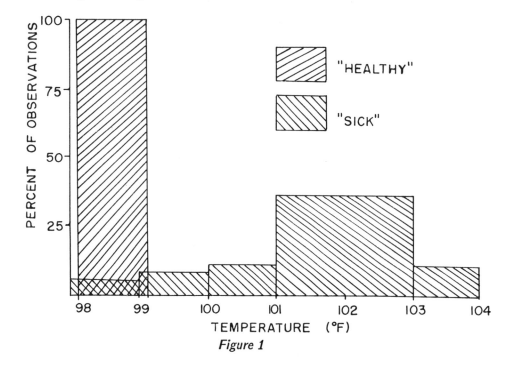

Figure 1

In this instance the single measurement temperature is the index; the higher the temperature, the more serious the illness. We could also use the index to define "illness." That is, we could say that a patient is "ill" if the temperature is *not* between 98°F and 99.1°F.

This index is simple but probably entailed a great deal of research time and data in its development.

Indices of injury severity are more difficult to develop. Response to serious injury can be very complicated. Such an index and the method of its development are described in the following section.

C. Trauma Score — An Index of Injury Severity

The Trauma Score is a measure of injury severity. It is based on seven assessments[1] that doctors, nurses, or paramedics can obtain easily. These assessments were selected from among 16 considered originally.

The seven assessments are:

- respiratory rate
- respiratory effort
- capillary refill
- systolic blood pressure
- eye-opening
- best verbal response
- best motor response.

The method for going from assessments to the computation of the Trauma Score is given in Table 1.

Eye-opening, best verbal response, and best motor response also make up the Glasgow Coma Scale, itself an index. The Glasgow Coma Scale is used worldwide as an index of injury to the central nervous system, which includes the brain and spinal cord.

EXAMPLE. Suppose an accident victim had the following assessments and codes:

Measurement	Assessment	Code
A. Respiratory Rate	12	A. 4
B. Respiratory Effort	Normal	B. 1
C. Systolic Blood Pressure	127	C. 4
D. Capillary Refill	Normal	D. 2
E. Based on Glasgow Coma Scale		E. 5
	Total	16
1. Eye-opening	Spontaneous	4
2. Verbal Response	Oriented	5
3. Motor Response	Obeys Commands	6
	Glasgow Coma Scale	15

The Trauma Score for this patient is $A+B+C+D+E = 16$. In this example the Glasgow Coma Scale is 15, so $E = 5$. (See Table 1.)

---

[1] Appendix II contains complete definitions for the assessments. You are urged to read these to familiarize yourself with the terminology.

Table 1
Trauma Score
Variable Definitions, Methods of Assessment, and Codes

	Rate	Codes	Score
A. Respiratory Rate	10–24	4	
Number of respirations in 15 seconds;	25–35	3	
multiply by four	≥36	2	
	1–9	1	
	0	0	A. _____
B. Respiratory Effort			
Shallow — Markedly decreased chest movement or air exchange	Normal	1	
Retractive — Use of accessory muscles	Shallow or Retractive	0	B. _____
C. Systolic Blood Pressure			
Systolic cuff pressure — either arm	≥ 90	4	
	70–89	3	
	50–69	2	
	1–49	1	
No pulse	0	0	C. _____
D. Capillary Refill			
Normal — Nail bed color refill in 2 seconds	Normal	2	
Delayed — More than 2 seconds capillary refill	Delayed	1	
None — No capillary refill	None	0	D. _____

E. Glasgow Coma Scale

1. Eye Opening

Spontaneous	_____4
To Voice	_____3
To Pain	_____2
None	_____1

2. Verbal Response

Oriented	_____5
Confused	_____4
Inappropriate Words	_____3
Incomprehensible Sounds	_____2
None	_____1

3. Motor Response

		Total GCS Points	Score
Obeys Commands	_____6		
Purposeful Movements (pain)	_____5		
Withdraw (pain)	_____4	14–15	5
Flexion (pain)	_____3	11–13	4
Extension (pain)	_____2	8–10	3
None	_____1	5–7	2
		3–4	1

Total GCS point (1 + 2 + 3)_____   E._____

Trauma Score
(Total Points $A + B + C + D + E$)_____

The following assessments have been made on 4 patients.[2] Find the Trauma Score for each patient.

PATIENT	1	2	3	4
Respiratory Rate	40	7	0	15
Respiratory Effort	Shallow	Retractive	Shallow	Normal
Systolic Blood Pressure	100	65	0	120
Capillary Refill	Delayed	Delayed	None	Normal
Eye-opening	To voice	To pain	None	Spontaneous
Verbal Response	Confused	Inappropriate Words	None	Oriented
Motor Response	Purposeful Movement	Flexion	None	Obeys Commands
TRAUMA SCORE	9.____	10. ____	11.____	12. ____

Table 2 contains data from trauma patients seen at Washington Hospital Center, Washington, D.C. The assessments were made by nurses when the patients arrived at the hospital by helicopter or ambulance. The number of patients varies because some assessments were not obtained on some patients.

Using Table 2, determine:

13. The number of patients with systolic blood pressure assessments. ____

14. The number of survivors and the number of deaths among the 1924 patients with Glasgow Coma Scale assessments.
   a. Number of survivors? _____
   b. Number of deaths? _____

15. The number of survivors and the number of deaths in the delayed category for capillary refill.
   a. Number of survivors? _____
   b. Number of deaths? _____

16. The fraction of survivors among the patients with capillary refill assessments. _____

---

[2] These might be thought of as 4 patients who were removed from the rubble of a collapsed building after the earthquake.

Note 1: Your answer to Problem 16 should be 1548/1714 or about .90 to the nearest hundredth.[3] The numerator (1548) is the number of survivors and the denominator (1714) is the total number of patients with capillary refill assessments.

Note 2: This fraction, for a given patient set, is sometimes called the "prior" probability of survival and is denoted by the symbol P. For a patient set,

$$P = \text{Number of Survivors/Total Number of Patients}$$

Table 2
PROBABILITY OF SURVIVAL ESTIMATES
FOR EACH ASSESSMENT OF EACH ADMISSION VARIABLE

Variable	Assessment	Number in Category	Number of Survivors	Number of Deaths	Fraction of Total Patients	Probability of Survival, P_s
Respiratory Effort (1839 Patients)	Normal	1501	1471	30	0.82	0.98
	Shallow/ Retractive	237	192	45	0.13	0.81
	None	101	9	92	0.054	0.089
	TOTALS		1672	167		
Capillary Refill (1714 Patients)[4]	Immediate (Normal)	1433	1400	33	0.84	0.98
	Delayed	281	148	133	0.16	0.53
	TOTALS		1548	166		
Glasgow Coma scale (1924 Patients)	(3,4)	144	26	118	0.075	0.18
	(5,6,7)	37	25	12	0.019	0.68
	(8,9,10)	49	37	12	0.025	0.76
	(11,12,13)	75	67	8	0.039	0.89
	(14,15)	1619	1594	25	0.84	0.98
	TOTALS		1749	175		
Systolic Blood Pressure (2780 Patients)	0	101	10	91	0.036	0.10
	1–49	9	4	5	0.003	0.44
	50–69	39	25	14	0.014	0.64
	70–89	92	79	13	0.033	0.86
	≥ 90	2539	2465	74	0.91	0.97
	TOTALS		2583	197		
Respiratory Rate (2622 Patients)	0	113	10	103	0.043	0.088
	1–9	7	2	5	0.003	0.286
	10–24	2119	2082	37	0.808	0.98
	25–35	306	287	19	0.117	0.94
	≥ 36	77	69	8	0.029	0.90
	TOTALS		2450	172		

[3] Many computations are requested in the monograph. Use all available figures in your computations and write your final answer to the nearest hundredth or two significant digits.

[4] Note that in this data set, all patients fell into the first two categories of capillary refill assessments.

Find the following:

17. Prior probability of survival values for the patient sets of the 4 other variables.

Variable	P Value
Respiratory Effort	a. _____
Glasgow Coma Scale	b. _____
Systolic Blood Pressure	c. _____
Respiratory Rate	d. _____

18. The fraction of patients in the delayed category for capillary refill. ____

    Note: Your answer to Problem 18 should be .16, which is the decimal equivalent of 281/1714.

19. The fraction of survivors among patients in the immediate (normal) category for capillary refill. _____

    Note: Your answer to Problem 19 should be .98, which is the decimal equivalent of 1400/1433.

    We call this quantity the probability of survival, P_S. The P_S values appear in the last column of Table 2. It is not surprising that the P_S values differ from P values because the P_S values are obtained on a subset of patients.

20. Find the probability of survival for patients in the delayed category for capillary refill. _____

21. Which variable "seems" to be the best for predicting survival and death?

    _____

    The worst? _____

22. Using your judgement, rank the 5 variables from best to worst with respect to the prediction of survival and death.

                                  VARIABLE

Best	_____
Next	_____
Next	_____
Next	_____
Worst	_____

23. Can you explain your rationale for the ranking? _____

    _____
    _____
    _____
    _____

Actually this question is difficult to answer with the information we have. Systolic blood pressure and respiratory rate involve the highest percentage of survivors, but we don't know how well they predicted which individual patients survived or died.

There are several ways of measuring the predictive capability of a variable. One powerful method called "relative information gain" is now illustrated using the data for capillary refill.

D. Information Gain

Recall that 1548 of 1714 patients survived in the data set for capillary refill and that

$$P = 1548/1714 = 0.90.$$

Given no information concerning a patient from this set, .90 represents the best estimate of his probability of survival. The power of capillary refill as a predictor can be thought of as being the average change in the estimate of probability of survival when you are given the assessment of capillary refill of a particular patient.

For most of these patients (0.84 or 84%) the assessment of capillary refill is "immediate," and after obtaining such a response, we would alter the estimate of probability of survival from $P = 0.90$ to $P_s(\text{immediate}) = 0.98$, a change of 0.08.

For the remaining patients (.16 or 16%) the assessment is "delayed," and after obtaining that response, we would alter the estimate of probability of survival from $P = .90$ to $P_s(\text{delayed}) = .53$, a change of .37. Since 84 out of every 100 persons are in the immediate category, while only 16 out of every 100 persons are in the delayed category, the changes in these categories must be weighted by .84 and .16. Therefore, "on the average" the change is

$$.84(.08) + .16(.37) = .13.$$

This average change is called the "information gain" and denoted by E. (*Note*: We used absolute value since we are interested in the amount of change and not whether it was higher or lower.) We can rewrite the expression for E in symbols, which will help to understand how E would be computed for other variables.

.84 = fraction of total patients with "immediate" observation for capillary refill. Denote as $f(\text{immediate})$.

.08 = change in the estimate of probability of survival from P to the probability of survival for all patients with capillary refill of "immediate." Denote as $|P - P_s(\text{immediate})|$ where $|\quad|$ means absolute value.

Similarly, .16 and .37 can be denoted as $f(\text{delayed})$ and $|P - P_s(\text{delayed})|$, respectively. Therefore, E can be written as:

$$E = f(\text{immediate}) \cdot |P - P_s(\text{immediate})| + f(\text{delayed}) \cdot |P - P_s(\text{delayed})|.$$

The calculation of E was explained by using capillary refill as an example of a variable that can take on only two "values," "immediate" and "delayed." But how is E calculated for variables which can take on many values?

Consider a variable x which can take on a wide range of values. Suppose this range is divided into 5 intervals. Let P, as before, be the prior probability of survival. Let f_i and $P_s(i)$ be defined for interval $i = 1, 2, 3, 4,$ and 5 as:

f_i = the fraction of total patients whose value of x falls into interval i;

and

$P_s(i)$ = the fraction of survivors among patients whose value of x is in interval i.

Then E is computed by the following formula

$$E = f_1|P - P_s(1)| + f_2|P - P_s(2)| + f_3|P - P_s(3)| \\ + f_4|P - P_s(4)| + f_5|P - P_s(5)|.$$

Of course, the formula extends to any number of intervals chosen.

Consider the variable "age." It is a measurement which is routinely obtained. Further, it has in certain instances (e.g., for burn patients) been shown to be a useful predictor of patient survival. It may also be useful for the general population of severely injured persons. The data collected for "age" are shown in Table 3.

Table 3

i	Age Interval (1857 Patients)	Number in Category	Fraction of Total Patients f_i	Number of Survivors	Number of Deaths	Probability of Survival, P_s
1	0–15	42	0.023	42	0	1.00
2	16–30	648	0.35	616	32	0.95
3	31–50	582	0.31	557	25	0.96
4	51–60	215	0.12	207	8	0.96
5	61–70	176	0.095	166	10	0.94
6	71–80	128	0.069	122	6	0.95
7	81–90	59	0.032	50	9	0.85
8	91–100	7	0.0038	7	0	1.00
TOTALS		1857		1767	90	

We can now use the formula given earlier to calculate the information gain, E, for "age." There is one difference, however. In this example we have 8 intervals, and so the expression for E is

$$E = f_1|P - P_s(1)| + f_2|P - P_s(2)| + \cdots + f_8|P - P_s(8)|.$$

24. Calculate P for the "age" data set. (Recall that P is simply the fraction of the total number of patients with this measurement who survived.)

$$P = \underline{\hspace{4cm}}$$

25. Calculate E for the "age" data set

$$E = \rule{4cm}{0.4pt}$$

A direct comparison of the information gains, E values, for capillary refill and age may not be fair. You may notice that capillary refill was measured on 1714 patients while age was obtained from 1857 patients. Further, both measurements may have been obtained on few of the same patients, and little basis for comparison may exist. Suppose, for example, that all patients for whom capillary refill was recorded actually died.

26. What would the information gain, E, be for capillary refill, if the data base for that measurement contained *no* survivors?

$$E = \rule{4cm}{0.4pt}$$

In this instance, capillary refill does not aid, at all, in the prediction of patient outcome. Yet on data collected from another set of patients, containing both surviving and nonsurviving patients, capillary refill may prove to be a very powerful predictor. What is needed is some way to use the information gain, E, which will allow direct comparisons to be made for measurements obtained from different sets of patients. This leads us to the topic of Relative Information Gain.

E. **Relative Information Gain**

Let us compare the information gain for any measurement, say capillary refill, with that available from a "perfect predictor" *for the data set for that measurement.* A perfect predictor would change the estimate from P to 1.0 (certain survival) for all patients who will survive. Also a perfect predictor would change the probability of survival from P to 0 (certain death) for those patients who will die.

Suppose that another data set for capillary refill is found. In this instance, the variable is seen to be a perfect predictor. That is, survivors occur when and only when their capillary refill is immediate, and nonsurvivors occur when and only when a delayed refill occurs, as shown in this table.

Assessment	Number in Category	Fraction of Total Patients	Number of Survivors	Number of Deaths	Probability of Survival, P_S
Immediate	1433	1433/1704	1433	0	1
Delayed	281	281/1704	0	281	0
TOTALS	1704		1433	281	

According to our formula, the calculation of E is shown below.

$$E = f(\text{immediate}) \cdot |P - P_S(\text{immediate})| + f(\text{delayed}) \cdot |P - P_S(\text{delayed})|.$$

But because for this data set "immediate" equals survival and "delayed" equals death, the equation above changes to:

$$E = P \cdot |P - 1| + (1 - P) \cdot |P - 0|$$
$$= P \cdot (1 - P) + (1 - P) \cdot P$$
$$= 2P \cdot (1 - P).$$

Thus the information gain for a perfect predictor is:

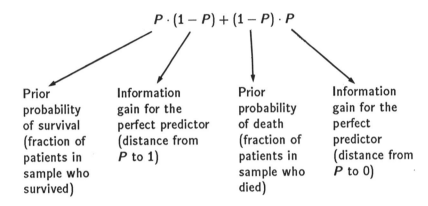

$$P \cdot (1 - P) + (1 - P) \cdot P$$

| Prior probability of survival (fraction of patients in sample who survived) | Information gain for the perfect predictor (distance from P to 1) | Prior probability of death (fraction of patients in sample who died) | Information gain for the perfect predictor (distance from P to 0) |

or

$$2P \cdot (1 - P).$$

For the original capillary refill data set, $P = .90$ and

$$2P \cdot (1 - P) = (1.80) \cdot (10) = .18.$$

One measure of how good capillary refill is as a predictor is the ratio of the information gain of capillary refill divided by the information gain of a perfect predictor:

$$R = \frac{E}{2P \cdot (1 - P)} = \frac{.13}{.18} = .72.$$

The R value is called the relative information gain. It reflects how good a predictor is relative to a perfect predictor. R takes on values from 0 to 1. The closer R is to 1, the better the predictor.

We have in previous exercises computed all entries for the table below, except R for age. Compute that quantity now.

27.

Age	Capillary Refill
$P = \underline{.95}$	$P = \underline{.90}$
$E = \underline{.0097}$	$E = \underline{.13}$
$R = \underline{}$	$R = \underline{.72}$

28. Which of the two variables, *age* or *capillary refill*, is most powerful as a predictor? _____

29. The value of which variable P, E, or R should be used as a basis for such a comparison? _____

Consider the data for the following variable X, which takes on values 1, 2, and 3.

Data for Measurement X

X Value	No. of Survivors	No. of Deaths	$P_s(X)$
1	16	16	.5
2	9	9	.5
3	4	4	.5
TOTALS	29	29	

30. Calculate P, E, and R for this variable and data set:

$P =$ _____

$E =$ _____

$R =$ _____

$R = 0$ because $P_s(X) = P$ for each value of X. Hence, the variable X gives no new information over that provided by P.

31. Consider the following data for the measurement Y, which also takes on the values 1, 2, and 3. Please fill in entries for the fourth column.

Data for Measurement Y

Y Value	No. of Survivors	No. of Deaths	Decimal Fraction of Total Patients	$P_s(Y)$
1	20	0	_____	1.0
2	10	10	_____	0.5
3	0	10	_____	0.0
TOTALS	30	20		

32. Compute P, E, and R for this variable, Y, and data set:

$P =$ _____

$E =$ _____

$R =$ _____

The computed R value should be $.67 = .32/.48$. The predicting power of Y is better than that of X because knowing the value of Y for a specific patient significantly improves your ability to make a correct estimate of the probability of survival when compared to the estimate provided by P. The measurement X provides no such information.

33. Now consider the variable Z, which also takes on the values 1, 2, and 3. Fill in the table given below so that the computed value of R will be 1.0 — that is, so that Z is a perfect predictor of outcome. Assume a total of 50 patients.

Data for Measurement Z

Z Value	No. of Survivors	No. of Deaths	$P_S(Z)$
1	_____	_____	____
2	_____	_____	____
3	_____	_____	____
TOTALS	_____	_____	____

Now you know how a mathematician might evaluate the predictive power of the individual variables. Such a process usually yields a much smaller set of very useful variables which can be used to construct an index. This approach was used to discard several of the 16 variables originally considered for use in the Trauma Score. Recall that the final Trauma Score uses only 7 variables or assessments.

If a single variable is powerful enough to be used alone as an index, the construction is rather simple. For example, capillary refill provides the following "index" or way to estimate probability of survival:

Assessment	Probability of Survival
Immediate	.98
Delayed	.53

But recall that the relative information gain of capillary refill is only 72% of that available from a perfect predictor.

Perhaps one of the other 4 assessments is better.

34. Using the data from Table 2, page 6, compute information gains and relative information gains for:

Respiratory Expansion _____

Glasgow Coma Scale _____

Respiratory Rate _____

Systolic Blood Pressure _____

35. Using R values, rank the 5 variables from best to worst.

VARIABLE

Best _____

Next _____

Next _____

Next _____

Worst _____

36. Do these rankings compare favorably with the rankings of Problem 22?

_____

The best single measurement is the Glasgow Coma Scale with an R value of 0.74. This is only slightly better than capillary refill.

The Trauma Score is one attempt to improve the predictions by combining the 5 variables as a simple sum $A+B+C+D+E$. Table 4 contains probability of survival estimates for the Trauma Score based on 1721 patients, 1542 of whom survived.

37. Compute E and R for the Trauma Score.

E: _____ R: _____

The Trauma Score is more powerful than any of the individual variables.

Table 4
Probability of Survival Estimates
for Each Value of the Trauma Score

Trauma Score	Total Number of Patients	Fraction of Patients	Number of Survivors	Probability of Survival, P_s
16	1017	0.59	1009	0.992
15	274	0.16	269	0.982
14	122	0.071	116	0.951
13	65	0.038	61	0.938
12	43	0.025	36	0.837
11	28	0.016	18	0.643
10	32	0.019	19	0.594
9	10	0.0058	5	0.500
8	10	0.0058	5	0.500
7	7	0.0041	1	0.143
6	12	0.0070	1	0.083
5	3	0.0017	0	0.000
4	7	0.0041	0	0.000
3	2	0.0012	0	0.000
2	89	0.052	2	0.022
1	0	0.000	0	–
TOTALS	1721		1542	

F. Tying Up Loose Ends

You may be uneasy, as we were, with some of the data and methods used so far. In particular, two weaknesses stand out. The first weakness is apparent from sparse data in Trauma Scores 3 to 9 in Table 4.

This leads to unlikely results such as the same probability of survival estimates for Trauma Scores of 8 and 9 and a much lower estimate for a Trauma Score of 7.

For example, if the next two patients who are assessed have Trauma Scores of 8, and they both die, the P_s for Trauma Score 8 would change from 0.500 to 0.417 and would be lower than the P_s for Trauma Score 9. However, if these patients both survived, the P_s for Trauma Score 8 would be 0.583 — higher than the P_s for Trauma Score 9. Small changes in data result in large changes in P_s estimates. This is not desirable.

The second possible weakness is that the Trauma Score does not give greater importance to more powerful assessments. It is a simple sum $A + B + C + D + E$ of the assessments; that is, each term in the sum is given the same weight, namely 1.

We now introduce a powerful method, the so-called logistic function, which is often used to address both weaknesses. It is used to represent data and provide more sensible and robust[5] results for the problem of sparse data. This method can be used to assign weights to the assessments, in a way which takes into account the predictive power of each assessment. We will demonstrate the utility of the logistic function by applying it to the Trauma Score data given earlier.

G. **Representing Data by the Logistic Function**

To represent the probability of survival data of Table 4, we write the logistic function:

$$P_S(W) = \frac{1}{1 + e^{-W}} \, .$$

where

$Ps(W) =$ an estimate of the probability of survival associated with W;

$e =$ the base of the natural logarithm system,

$W = w_0 + w_1 \cdot (\text{Trauma Score}).$

The quantities w_0 and w_1 are numbers (called weights) which are to be determined from the data of Table 4. The process for determining these weights is called "curve fitting."

See Appendix III for more information about curve fitting.

38. Use your calculator (or mathematics tables)[6] to evaluate $P_S(W)$ for

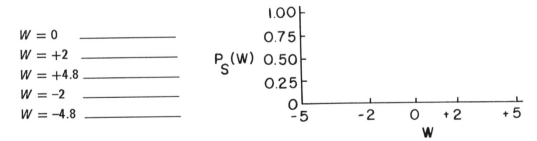

$W = 0$ _____

$W = +2$ _____

$W = +4.8$ _____

$W = -2$ _____

$W = -4.8$ _____

Plot the computed values on the axes provided.

Can you find a value of W so that $P_s(W) > 1.0$?

---

[5] By robust we mean that the results will be less dependent on small changes in the data.

[6] If tables are unavailable, spend several minutes reviewing the answers we have provided. If your calculator does not have an "e^x" key, then store the value of $e = 2.71828$ and use the y^x key.

Returning to the Trauma Score, Figure 2 is a plot of the (Trauma Score, Probability of Survival) data of Table 4.

The objective of the "curve fitting" is to find values of the weights in the equation so that the resulting equation is a good representation of the data. In this example our equation is:

$$P_S(T) = \frac{1}{1 + e^{-(w_0 + w_1 \cdot T)}} \ .$$

where T is the Trauma Score.

Let's try to guess values of w_0 and w_1. We observe from the previous equation that

$$P_S(T) = 1/2 \quad \text{if} \quad w_0 + w_1 \cdot T = 0.$$

Also a T of 9 is associated with a 50% survival rate from the data. Therefore we let

$$w_0 + 9w_1 = 0.$$

Also presuming that the curve will fit well for $T = 16$ we have

$$\underset{\underset{P_S(W)}{\uparrow}}{.992} \quad = \quad \frac{1}{1 + \underset{\underset{W = w_0 + 16w_1}{\uparrow}}{e^{-W}}}$$

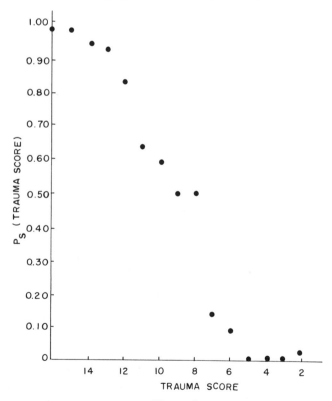

Figure 2

We have to guess a value of W (with the help of a calculator) that leads to a value of 0.992 for $P_s(W)$. Better yet, consult the answer to Problem 38 for $W = 4.8$. We see that $P_s(4.8)$ is approximately 0.992.

Solving the two equations

$$w_0 + 9w_1 = 0, \tag{1}$$

$$w_0 + 16w_1 = 4.8 \tag{2}$$

for w_0 and w_1, we get

$$w_0 = -6.174$$

$$w_1 = 0.686.$$

These are estimates of the weights.

A computer program was also used to estimate the weights based on iterative methods. By iterative we mean guess — evaluate the fit — change the guess — re-evaluate the fit, and so on. The details of the algorithm are not important to you at this stage. However, the estimates were not too different from yours. The values were $w_0 = -6.5432$ and $w_1 = 0.702$. Hence the logistic function for the Trauma Score data is

$$P_s(T) = \frac{1}{1 + e^{-(-6.5432 + 0.702\,T)}}.$$

Figure 3 contains a comparison of the original estimates and the smoothed estimates based on the logistic function.

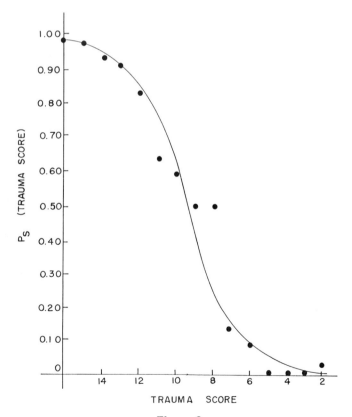

Figure 3

H. Application of Logistic Function to Weighted Assessment

You will recall that the Trauma Score is actually computed from the values of 5 variables — respiratory rate, respiratory effort, systolic blood pressure, capillary refill, and the Glasgow Coma Scale. The logistic function can be used to relate probability of survival to the values of one or more measurements, e.g.,

$$P_S = \frac{1}{1 + e^{-(w_0 + w_1 A + w_2 B + \cdots + w_5 E)}}.$$

Thus, we could have used the logistic function to derive the weights (w's) for each of the 5 measurements which make up the Trauma Score. In fact, we did just that! However, the accuracy of the predictions differed only slightly from those obtained with the Trauma Score. Hence the simple sum form of the Trauma Score was adopted because of its simplicity and power.

Part II
APPLICATIONS OF THE TRAUMA SCORE TO TRIAGE AND SORTING OF PATIENTS

A. Triage

Paramedics must make triage decisions quickly and accurately to determine if a patient requires the care provided by a specialized Trauma Center rather than standard hospital care. Trauma Centers are special facilities with extensive resources (general surgeons, thoracic surgeons, neurosurgeons, orthopedic surgeons, X-rays, CAT scans, blood banks,...) which are available, every day, at all hours, for the treatment of seriously injured patients.

A simple triage rule is

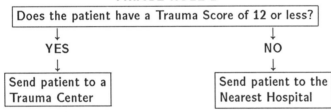

TRIAGE RULE 1

Does the patient have a Trauma Score of 12 or less?

↓   ↓

YES   NO

↓   ↓

Send patient to a Trauma Center	Send patient to the Nearest Hospital

The objective of triage is to identify patients with high risk of dying from their injuries. Once identified, these patients should be sent to the level of care which can adequately treat their injuries and hopefully increase their chances of survival. A more realistic proposed triage rule follows. Some of the information that it calls for is not always available. In such cases, of course, the triage decision must be made with the information that is available.

TRIAGE RULE 2

Patients with any of the following should be taken to the nearest trauma center:

1. **Mechanism of Blunt Injury**
   a. Patients involved in high-speed (greater than 40 mph) moving vehicular accidents
   b. Patients hit by vehicles moving at greater than 20 mph
   c. Patients thrown from vehicles
   d. Patients falling from heights greater than 20 feet

2. **Location of Penetrating Injury**
   a. Patients with penetrating injury to head, neck, chest, abdomen, pelvis, or groin

3. **Location of Blunt (Nonpenetrating) Injury**
   a. Blunt injury with significant involvement of a single body system
   b. Any multiple system injury
   c. Two or more proximal long bone fractures

4. **Physiological Distress**

   A degree of respiratory distress, shock, or coma that results in a Trauma Score of 12 or less or a Glasgow Coma Scale of 10 or less

Table 5

Probability for Survival Estimates
for Each Value of the Trauma Score

1509   Patients (Blunt and Penetrating)
139   Deaths

Trauma Score (i)	Fraction of Total Patients	Probability of Survival, $P_s(i)$
16	0.64	0.99
15	0.16	0.98
14	0.064	0.96
13	0.037	0.93
12	0.023	0.87
11	0.013	0.76
10	0.015	0.60
9	0.0053	0.42
8	0.0040	0.26
7	0.0033	0.15
6	0.0066	0.08
5	0.0013	0.04
4	0.0033	0.02
3	0.0013	0.01
2	0.044	0.00
1	0	0.00

39. Using Table 5, estimate the fraction of patients that would be sent to a Trauma Center by TRIAGE RULE 1. _____

40. Would more patients be sent to a trauma center by RULE 1 or RULE 2?

_____

Paramedics at the scene of a four-car accident find 6 victims with the following diagnoses and assessments.

Victim	Injury Diagnosis	Glasgow Coma Scale	Trauma Score
1	Broken arm	15	14
2	Head and chest contusions (bruises)	8	13
3	No obvious injuries	10	13
4	Abdominal contusion	15	12
5	Abdominal contusion	15	16
6	Fractured cheekbone	11	13

41. According to RULE 2, which victims would be sent to a trauma center?

_____

B. **Sorting**

Sorting is the cornerstone for handling mass casualties in order to provide the greatest benefit for the largest number of patients. This example of a proposed simple sorting rationale, for civilian or military mass casualty situations, uses the Trauma Score. The goal of the sorting is to maximize the expected number of survivors.

Step 1: A physician or specially trained nurse or paramedic sorts the casualties into several categories including:
   A. Those who will survive with little or no medical assistance;
   B. Those who have virtually no chance of survival even with the best possible care;
   C. Those who will survive only if they receive substantial medical care.

Step 2: The casualties in Category C are ranked using the probability of survival, P_s, based on the Trauma Score; the higher the patient's P_s, the sooner he or she is treated.

To use this rationale, a sorter must be capable of obtaining a Trauma Score on a patient and must have the table of probabilities of survival, which could be put on a 3×5 inch card. Now that you are familiar with triage and sorting and their implications for saving lives, let's return to our disaster scenario, with an added bulletin at 2:00 P.M.

10:00 A.M.

Thirty minutes ago, the city of San Francisco was nearly leveled by the major earthquake scientists have been predicting for the last few years. The quake measured 7.8 on the Richter Scale, with an epicenter only 10 miles outside the heavily populated city.

An estimate of property damage is about 200 billion dollars. No estimate is yet available for loss of life.

The President has declared the area a Disaster Area, and the Red Cross is mobilizing all of its resources to help. Citizens in the area have been warned to boil all water for consumption because of contamination.

Hospitals in the area that are still able to function are swamped with victims. Those injured who are able to are requested to wait 24 hours before attempting to enter the emergency rooms.

All physicians and other medical personnel in the area are requested to report to the nearest hospital to help with the enormous number of injured victims.

2:00 P. M.

More news on the earthquake disaster. Medical officials have reported that there are about 1,000 seriously injured victims waiting for substantial medical care. These patients will probably not survive for 24 hours if the care is unavailable.

A team of 100 paramedics are assigned to assess the Trauma Scores of the 1,000 patients on a continuous basis. In the first assessment at 1400 hours, we have the following distribution of Trauma Scores.

Trauma Score i	Number of Victims with Trauma Score i	Probability of Survival, P_s, from smoothed data
12	400	.87
11	50	.76
10	50	.62
8	100	.28
6	100	.09
4	200	.02
2	100	.01

At 1400 hours, resources become available to treat 400 patients.

42. Which patients would you select for treatment? _____

_____

43. How many would you expect to survive? _____

_____

A medical officer, with no triage experience, selects for treatment the most seriously injured patients. Hence the care proceeds for victims with Trauma Scores of 6, 4, and 2. The resources are tied up until 1600 hours. Ten of these patients survive, all 10 of whom had Trauma Scores of 6.

By 1600 hours, 200 of the 600 waiting for treatment have died. The remaining 400 patients are reassessed as:

Trauma Score i	Number of Victims with Trauma Score i	Probability of Survival, P_s, from smoothed data
6	300	.09
2	100	.01

These 400 patients begin therapy at 1600 hours and 32 survive.

Altogether there were 42 survivors. If we had chosen to treat the less seriously injured patients first, the expected number of survivors would have been greater than 350.

Part III
PATIENT TRACKING

New technology has brought to the bedside of critically ill patients in intensive care and trauma centers a capability for monitoring life processes which previously existed only in the laboratory. With the new monitors has come an overwhelming accumulation of data, facts, and measurements that all too often leave the medical doctor in a quandary as to the meaning of all the numbers accumulated. That is, they have a great deal of *data* and very little information.

Many physicians have turned to the computer for help with the storage, retrieval, and display of patient data. Unfortunately, most medical computers merely display data for the doctor; they do not interpret the data nor tell the doctor how to use it to treat the patient. This situation is changing as a result of the research of several teams composed of physicians and mathematical scientists.

These teams have devoted considerable effort to distilling, from as many as 60 different physiological and biochemical variables, those which contain the most useful information. These surviving measurements are then incorporated into indices and mathematical models for tracking patients for the purpose of:

1. Estimating probability of survival as a function of time; and hence

2. Establishing patient trends;

3. Taking medical action;

4. Evaluating the effect of medical actions.

One such study resulted in the CHOP and Respiratory Indices, described in the following sections.

A. CHOP Index

The CHOP Index is based on 4 variables: serum creatinine (C), hematocrit (H), serum osmolality (O), and systolic blood pressure (P).[1]

These variables are important and powerful indicators for tracking a patient in an intensive care unit.

Take systolic blood pressure, denoted P, as an example. It is a measure of how strongly the heart is pumping. The average value for systolic blood pressure for healthy adults, usually written as $\overline{P}$, is 127.0 mmHg.[2] We call this the normal value. If a patient's systolic blood pressure is much higher or lower than 127.0, it could indicate a problem.

Consider the following formula for a blood pressure index,

$$P_D = |P - \overline{P}| = |P - 127.0|.$$

This index measures "difference from normal."

44. Find the value of P_D for the following patients.

Patient	P	P_D
1	75.0	_____
2	69.0	_____
3	0	_____
4	179.0	_____
5	254.0	_____
6	127.0	_____

Serum creatinine (C) is a waste product in the blood. When the kidneys are funtioning well, the level of creatinine is near 1.0, that is, $\overline{C} = 1.0$.

45. Find the difference measure $C_D = |C - \overline{C}|$ for the following patients.

Patient	C	C_D
1	1.0	_____
2	2.30	_____
3	4.20	_____
4	0.50	_____
5	8.00	_____

46. Find P_D and C_D for a patient with a systolic blood pressure of 137.0 and a serum creatinine of 5.0.

$$P_D = \text{_____}   ,   C_D = \text{_____}$$

---

[1] Many medical variables and special terms used in this section are defined in Appendix II.

[2] mmHg stands for millimeters of mercury, the usual units for measuring pressure.

We can represent this patient by a point in a (P_D, C_D) coordinate system as given below:

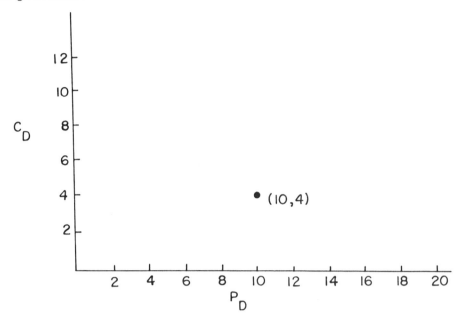

47. A patient with a creatinine value of _____ and a systolic blood pressure of _____ would be represented as a point at the *origin* in the (P_D, C_D) coordinate system.

48. Plot the points in the (P_D, C_D) coordinate system for patients 1–3. (Use the graph in Problem 46.)

Patient	Systolic Blood Pressure	Creatinine
1	147.0	2.0
2	120.0	3.0
3	130.0	5.0

Patient 3 (Problem 48) has coordinates (3,4) in the (P_D, C_D) system:

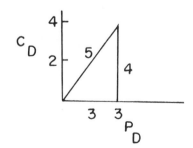

The distance of this point from the origin is (by the Pythagorean Theorem) $\sqrt{3^2 + 4^2}$ or 5. We can use this distance measure to combine P_D and C_D. If the distance measure is called D, then

$$D = \sqrt{P_D{}^2 + C_D{}^2}.$$

49. Compute D for patients 1 and 2 of Problem 48.

Patient	D
1	_____
2	_____

As you may have noticed, there are problems with using D as a "distance from normal." Since systolic blood pressure is a large number and creatinine is a small number, D is more influenced by systolic blood pressure.

As an example, for the patient with P, C values of 147.0 and 2.0,

$$D = \sqrt{P_D{}^2 + C_D{}^2} = \sqrt{20^2 + 1^2} = \sqrt{401} \approx 20.025.$$

So creatinine contributes little to D, even though a creatinine value of 2.0 is a much more serious symptom than a systolic blood pressure of 147.0.

To alleviate this problem, a procedure called *normalization* is used to make distance values more meaningful. As used here, *normalize* is a mathematical term rather than a medical one. The objective of normalization is to rate each component of the distance measure on a similar basis.

Consider the plots shown in Figures 4 and 5, which are based on data from survivors. The measurements were taken on the last day that the patients were in the intensive care unit.

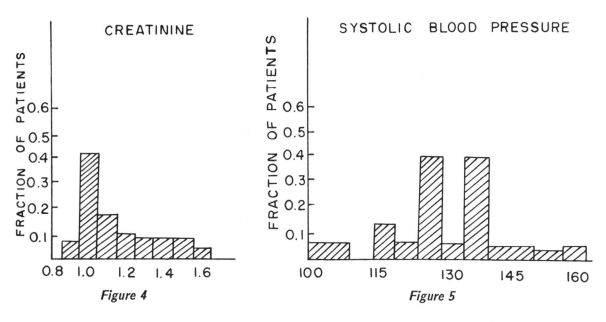

Figure 4   Figure 5

Mathematicians use many different statistical parameters to characterize the shape, size, and range of such distributions, including many terms you may be familiar with, such as *average* (or *mean*), *median*, and *mode*. A measure of spread that is often used is standard deviation. (The computation of standard deviation is described in Appendix V.)

With the average, $\overline{M}$, and the standard deviation, $S(M)$, available for any variable M, we have a way to *normalize* M consistently. The normalized value of M, call it M_n, is a representation of M *in standard deviation units from the average.*

In symbols,

$$M_n = \frac{M - \overline{M}}{S(M)}.$$

For systolic blood pressure, a reading of 169.0, then, gives

$$P_n = \frac{P - \overline{P}}{S(P)} = \frac{169 - 127}{21} = +2.0.$$

This +2.0 means that 169 is 2 standard deviations from the average.

Similarly, for creatinine, a reading of .25 gives

$$C_n = \frac{C - \overline{C}}{S(C)} = \frac{.25 - 1.0}{0.5} = -1.5.$$

This means that .25 is 1.5 standard deviations *less* than the average of 1.0.

50. Normalize the following readings of systolic blood pressure (P) and creatinine (C) and compute D_n.

Note 1: $\overline{P} = 127$, $S(P) = 21$, $\overline{C} = 1.0$, $S(C) = 0.5$.

Note 2: $D_n = \sqrt{P_n{}^2 + C_n{}^2}$.

Patient	P	P_n	C	C_n	D_n
1	148.0	_____	2.0	_____	_____
2	22.0	_____	1.0	_____	_____
3	253.0	_____	3.0	_____	_____
4	127.0	_____	5.0	_____	_____

For Patient 1 of the previous problem, $P = 148.0$, $C = 2.0$. Hence $P_n = 1.0$, $C_n = 2.0$, and $D_n = \sqrt{1^2 + 2^2}$. Thus, in contrast to our previous measure D, creatinine contributes more to D_n than systolic blood pressure. This is good news, because a creatinine value of 2.0 is more significant medically than a systolic blood pressure of 148.0.

The index D_n is called a *Euclidean distance measure.* As used here, D_n reflect the patient's "distance from normality" with respect to 2 measurements. $(D_n = 0$ means both measurements are equal to the normal average.)

The CHOP Index is an extension of the concept of D_n to 4 measurements, creatinine (C), hematocrit (H), osmolality (O), and systolic blood pressure (P). That is,

$$\text{CHOP Index} = \sqrt{C_n{}^2 + H_n{}^2 + O_n{}^2 + P_n{}^2},$$

where

$$C_n = \left(\frac{C - 1.0}{0.5}\right); \qquad \overline{C} = 1.0, \quad S(C) = 0.5$$

$$H_n = \left(\frac{H - 37.0}{6.0}\right); \qquad \overline{H} = 37.0, \quad S(H) = 6.0$$

$$O_n = \left(\frac{O - 292.0}{15.0}\right); \qquad \overline{O} = 292.0, \quad S(O) = 15.0$$

$$P_n = \left(\frac{P - 127.0}{21.0}\right); \qquad \overline{P} = 127.0, \quad S(P) = 21.0.$$

51. Compute the CHOP Index for the following patients.

Patient	C	H	O	P	CHOP Index
1	1.0	37.0	292.0	127.0	_____
2	3.0	25.0	322.0	64.0	_____
3	0.5	43.0	307.0	106.0	_____
4	6.0	13.0	367.0	43.0	_____

52. What would be the CHOP Index of a *perfectly* normal patient? _____

Given in Figure 6 is the CHOP Index "trajectory" of a 35-year-old male who died on day 7.

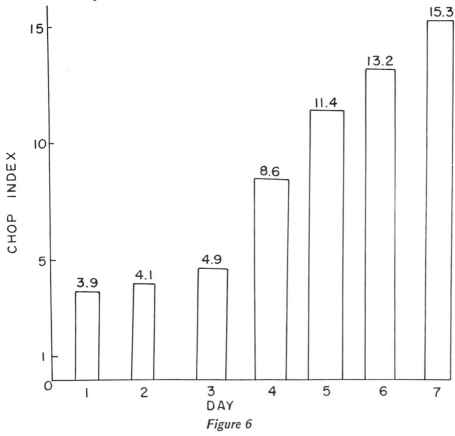

Figure 6

53. Compute the daily values of the CHOP Index of a 65-year-old male patient who died on day 5.

Day	C_n	H_n	O_n	P_n	CHOP Index
1	0.6	−0.8	1.7	−1.9	_____
2	1.2	−0.3	3.3	−2.4	_____
3	1.6	−0.3	4.0	−2.9	_____
4	0.2	−0.3	6.0	−3.3	_____
5	0.0	−0.7	5.3	−3.8	_____

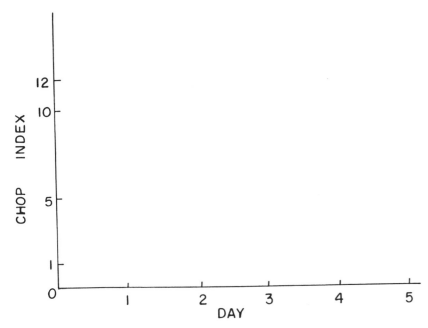

Plot the "trajectory" of this patient on the graph above as was done in Figure 6.

Table 6 contains CHOP Index data on 634 trauma patients who survived at least one day. When these data were "fit" (using the logistic function[3]) to patient outcome, the values of P_s given in the table were obtained[4].

Table 6

Peak (highest) value of the CHOP Index related to probability of survival (P_s) of 634 patients studied. Of these patients, 528 lived and 106 died. (Obtained with logistic function)

Peak CHOP Index Values	Probability of Survival, P_s
0–1.99	0.99
2.0–2.99	0.97
3.0–3.99	0.91
4.0–4.99	0.77
5.0–5.99	0.42
$\geq$ 6:0	0.14

54. What is the prior probability of survival P for the 634 patient data set?

Note: The definition of prior probability of survival is given after Problem 16.

---

[3] $P_s = 1/\left(1 + e^{-(w_0 + w_1 \cdot \text{CHOP Index})}\right)$

[4] While the logistic function can be used to obtain P_s for any value of peak CHOP Index, averages over the ranges in Table 6 were used for simplicity.

The relative information gain (R value) of the CHOP Index was 0.64 for this data set. Recall that this means it is 64% as good as a perfect index in predicting patient survival. The CHOP Index does not contain respiratory variables. To make predictions for patients with respiratory problems, a Respiratory Index was created. This index is described next.

B. Respiratory Index

In a healthy person the oxygen pressure of the blood in the lungs, O_L, equals the oxygen pressure of the blood in the arteries, O_A. Normally, $O_A = O_L = 100$ mmHg. The ratio $(O_L - O_A)/O_A$ is a measure of the respiratory condition; the bigger the ratio, the poorer the condition. O_L cannot be measured easily, but we can estimate it by $(713F - 35)$, where F is the fraction of oxygen in the "air" that is given to a patient from a ventilator or is equal to .20 when the patient is not on a ventilator, since room air contains about 20% oxygen. Hence the Respiratory Index, RI,[5] is the ratio

$$\frac{(713F - 35) - O_A}{O_A}.$$

55. Compute RI for the following patients:

Patient	O_A	F	RI
1	100	0.20	_____
2	37	0.20	_____
3	80	0.50	_____
4	40	0.80	_____

Male patient 1 has a normal O_A and is *not* on a ventilator. So he is breathing room air which contains 20% oxygen ($F = 0.20$). His RI is near zero.

The RI for female patient 2 is 1.9. She has a low O_A value and should be placed on a ventilator to get more oxygen. One goal of respiratory therapy is to keep O_A above 80.

Male patient 3 requires a high "dose" of oxygen ($F = .50$) to maintain an O_A of 80. An RI of 3.02 indicates that his respiratory condition is not good.

Even with $F = 0.80$, male patient 4 has a very low O_A value of 40. His condition is grave. His RI is over 12.

---

[5] See Appendix IV for a complete definition.

Table 7 contains Respiratory Index data from 177 trauma patients, 116 (66%) of whom survived. The RIs listed are the peak (maximal) RIs of the patients' entire hospital stay.

Table 7
Data For Respiratory Index

Peak Respiratory Index (RI)	Fraction of Total Patients	Probability of Survival, P_S
0–1	0.20	0.89
1.1–2	0.16	0.84
2.1–3	0.16	0.75
3.1–4	0.12	0.65
4.1–5	0.11	0.58
5.1–6	0.09	0.45
6.1 on	0.16	0.20

177 patients
116 survivors

56. The relative information gain (R value) for the Respiratory Index is

Respiratory Index Chart

We can use the Respiratory Index

$$RI = \frac{(713F - 35) - O_A}{O_A} \qquad (1)$$

to "track" a patient with respiratory problems, and to guide proper oxygen therapy.

Solve (1) for O_A.

$$O_A = \underline{\hspace{4cm}}$$

Your answer should be

$$O_A = \frac{713F - 35}{1 + RI}. \qquad (2)$$

For RI = 2,

$$O_A = \frac{713F - 35}{3}.$$

This is the equation of a line in the (F, O_A) coordinate system. Plot this line on the graph provided.

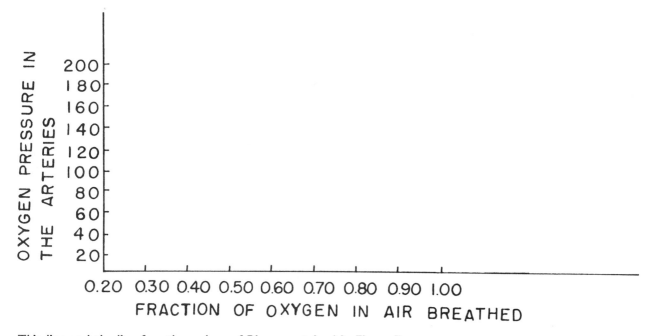

This line and the line for other values of RI are contained in Figure 7.

The letters *A, B, C* on the chart represent values of F and O_A for a male patient with chest injuries including 6 fractured ribs on the left side and bad lung contusions (bruises). Twenty minutes after the accident his O_A is 50, and he is breathing room air, so $F = 0.20$ (POINT A).

His RI is 1.0. He is then given 30% oxygen ($F = .30$) by "face mask." A repeat measurement of arterial oxygen shows an O_A of 55.

The RI is 2.0 (POINT B). His condition has worsened, calling for more drastic therapy. The patient was intubated. (By surgical operation a tube is inserted into the respiratory tract to assure a direct and clear airway through which oxygen can be administered.) The patient was given 40% oxygen ($F = 0.40$) through the tube using a mechanical respirator. The O_A increased to 120 and the RI improved to 1.0 (POINT C). The patient continued to improve and survived.

The letters *D* and *E* on the chart represent what "might have been." If the patient had gone from *C* to *D*, as a result of a decrease in O_A to 55, we could alter F from 0.40 to 0.60 hoping to slide the patient along the line (RI= 3) to *E*, because this would provide an increase in O_A to 95 (a much better condition). From that point on we would strive to keep O_A at 80 or above, while gradually reducing the oxygen levels to normal, because oxygen toxicity is a hazard when a patient is placed on high concentrations for long periods.

In summary, the chart can be used to track patients for respiratory problems and to provide guidelines for oxygen therapy.

RESPIRATORY INDEX

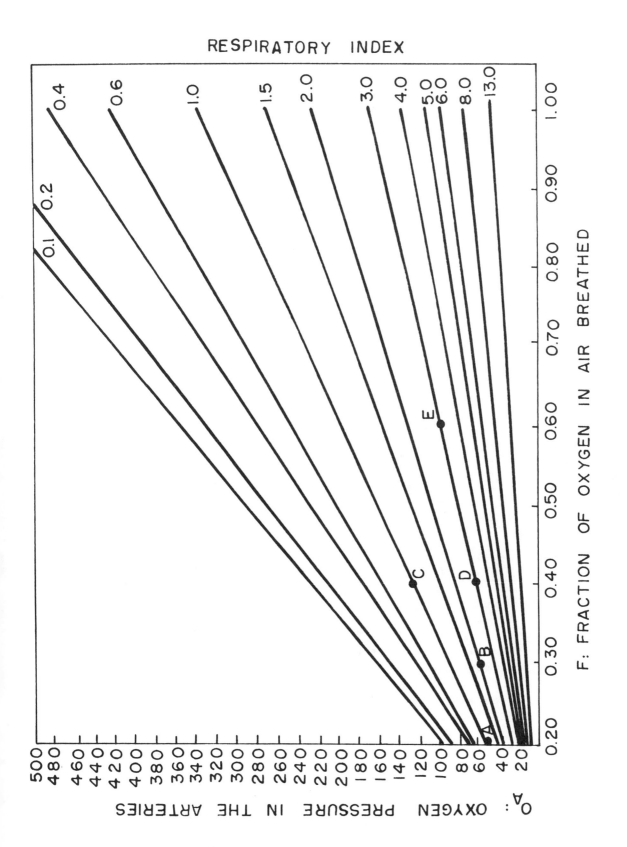

Figure 7

C. **Joint Use of CHOP and Respiratory Indices**

The CHOP and Respiratory Indices can be used together to improve predictive capabilities. Figure 8 is based on the same data set as Table 7. It contains regions A, B, C, D, each with an associated probability of survival, P_S, and fraction of patients F_A, F_B, F_C, F_D.

57. Compute the relative information gain (R value) for the CHOP–Respiratory Index pair.

$R = $ _____

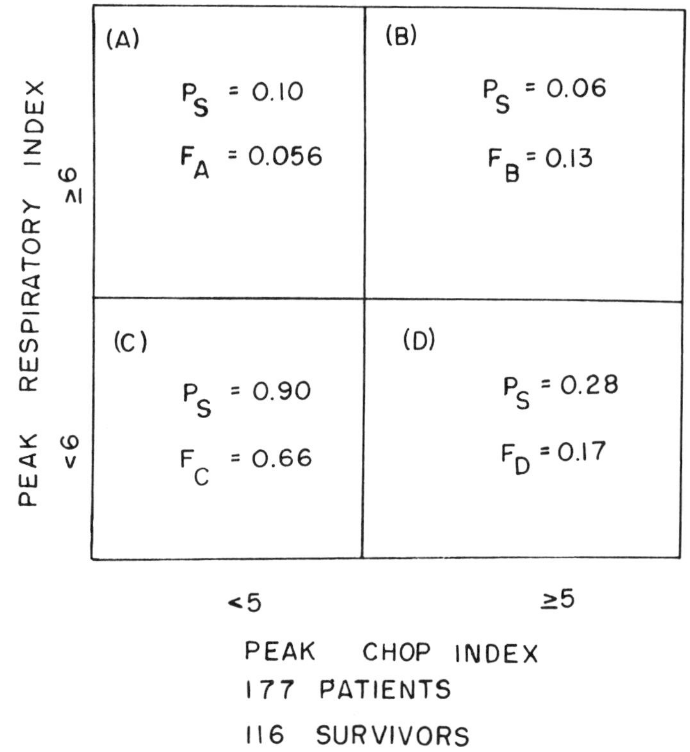

Figure 8

You can see the power of using two indices to predict the severity of patient illness by comparing the R value above to those for the CHOP and Respiratory Indices individually, which were 0.64 and 0.43, respectively.

Part IV
EVALUATION OF PATIENT CARE

The Trauma Score (TS) is used in combination with the Injury Severity Score to give a method by which an emergency department or a trauma center can evaluate the quality of care it provides to patients.

The Injury Severity Score (ISS) is another measure of patient injury. It is based solely on assessments of physical injuries like ruptured spleen, perforated liver, fractured ribs, or skull fracture. It takes on values from 1 to 75; the higher the score, the poorer the patient condition. Since the TS reflects the body's "response" to the injuries, together the ISS and the TS provide an accurate representation of injury severity.

This is illustrated in Figure 9. The points on the graph are TS–ISS pairs obtained from 218 consecutive serious trauma patients (automobile accidents and falls, mostly) seen at the Washington Hospital Center, Washington, D.C. The dots are for survivors; the x's are for deaths. Some patients have the same TS–ISS pair. These are indicated by a number near the point. Each point of the diagonal line has probability of survival of 0.50. This line is called the $P_S = 0.50$ *isobar*. Combinations of TS and ISS below the line have probabilities of survival greater that 0.50. Combinations above the line have probabilities of survival less than 0.50.

58. How many survivors are above the line? _____

59. How many deaths are below the line? _____

The set, S_A, of survivors above the line and the set, D_B, of deaths below the line are interesting patients for further review and study.

The patients in S_A may be success stories worthy of documentation and emulation. On the other hand, the patients in D_B may have benefited (in fact, are the patients most likely to have benefited) from alternative treatment. There are 7 patients in S_A and 8 patients in D_B. Thus a quality of care review immediately focuses on 15 patients, 6.8% of the patient population.

Figure 10 contains TS–ISS combinations from 201 trauma patients seen at a midwestern trauma center.

60. How many survivors are above the isobar? _____

61. How many deaths are below the isobar? _____

62. What per cent of the population qualifies for review using this method?

In summary this method identifies patients who appear to fall outside "normal" standards of care. It enables an emergency department or a trauma center to focus quickly on its strengths and shortcomings.

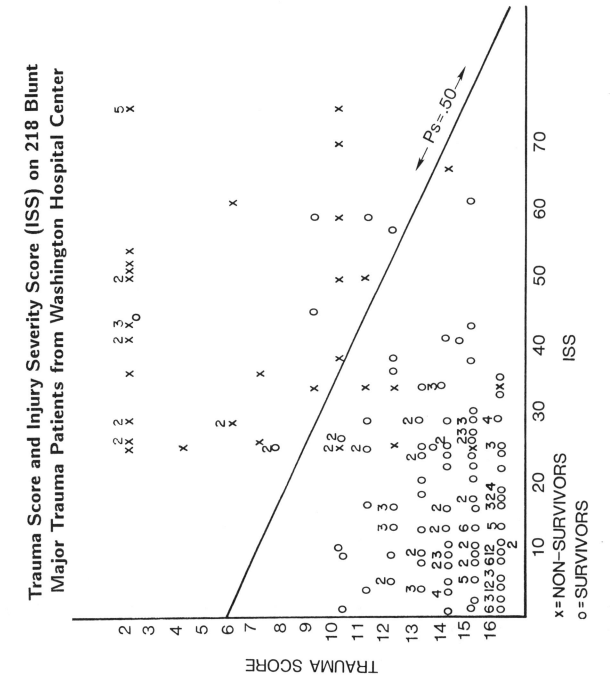

Figure 9

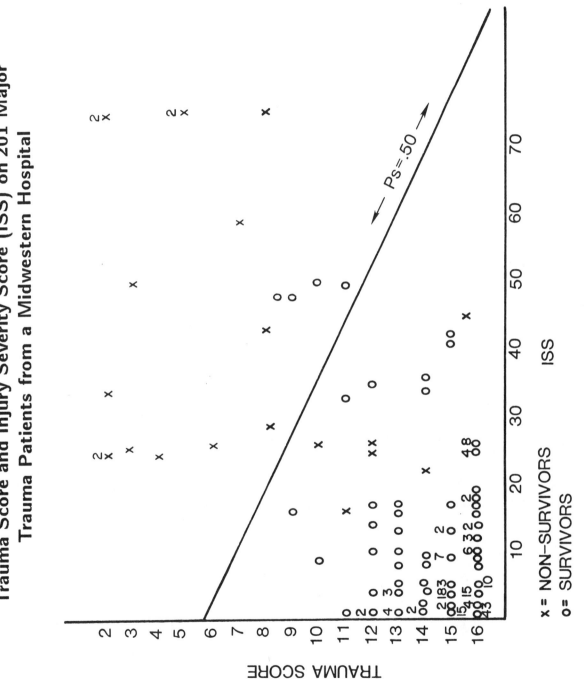

Trauma Score and Injury Severity Score (ISS) on 201 Major Trauma Patients from a Midwestern Hospital

Figure 10

Summary

In this monograph you have been given some information on indices: how common they are, techniques with which they can be derived, and examples of how they are being applied to real-world medical problems. Along the way you have also been exposed to some powerful and useful mathematical concepts and techniques such as relative information gain, curvefitting and the logistic function, normalization, and distance.

It is the hope of the authors that this material will give you a glimpse of one area where mathematics can be applied for the betterment of man.

Appendix I
DEFINITIONS AND EXAMPLES

Patient Triage

Triage is the decision made by the paramedic or ambulance driver as to where the accident victim(s) should be taken.

Is this really a big problem? Yes!

The nearby hospitals are not all at the same distance from the accident scene, so travel times may also be different. More importantly, hospitals are not all alike. Does the patient need a high-powered trauma (injury) center, a specialized burn center, or can his injuries be treated at an ordinary community hospital? The paramedic facing this problem needs better guidance than a simple rule to "Go to the nearest hospital." How does mathematics apply here? Should the ambulance crew crank up an on-board computer under the dashboard? No! What is needed is a standard, simple, and reliable procedure for judging the seriousness of the patient's injuries, which can be understood by all the ambulance crew and rehearsed many times in practice drills. The design of such a standard procedure should be guided by physicians, experienced in emergency medicine, with the help of applied mathematicians who collect, review, and analyze actual patient data and construct the simplest yet most powerful and reliable procedure possible.

Patient Sorting

The patient sorting problem arises in mass casualty situations. Suppose a huge earthquake strikes in Missouri. Unbelievable? There was a big one there in 1811. If it happened again, hospitals (the ones still standing) would be swamped with patients. The sorting problem is to identify patients with no chance of recovery so that doctors do not spend time on them and thereby lose the chance to save others.

Mass casualty situations come in all sizes from earthquake and military battles to the ten-car turnpike pileup, and even the "little" ones are enough to overload a local emergency care system.

Patient Tracking

In an intensive care unit, as many as 60 physiological and biochemical measurements are taken on each patient, many times a day. How can these measurements be used to assess: (1) a patient's condition, for example, the probability of survival; (2) the requirements for therapy; (3) the benefit gained from therapy given previously?

Again, mathematical scientists have been involved with physicians in selecting the powerful measurements and in developing graphic ways to "track" patients, that is, to mathematically monitor their progress (or lack of progress) during their treatment.

Evaluation of Patient Care

Many physicians believe that there are large differences in the quality of care provided by various treatment facilities. As a result, it may be that some patients die, who would have lived if treated in a different facility. Others want to know how the quality of care within one facility changes over time. How can such issues be evaluated? Again, mathematicians and statisticians are assisting in the development of the needed methods.

What do the techniques have in common? All are based on indices which measure the severity of patient illness or injury. In this monograph we describe the indices and their construction and use.

Appendix II
DEFINITIONS FOR THE VARIABLES
AND DESCRIPTIONS OF OTHER
MEDICAL TERMS

Respiratory Rate

Number of breaths per minute.

Respiratory Effort

Normal — Easily visible chest wall movement.

Shallow — Barely perceptible chest wall movement or air exchange.

Retractive — Chest wall movement that is assisted by any other muscles such as the neck muscles.

Systolic Blood Pressure

The health care professional records the blood pressure by using either the patient's right or left arm.

Capillary Refill

Capillary refill is assessed by firmly pressing a finger nail of a patient until the color disappears and the nail is white. The nail is then released and the time that passes until the color returns is assessed. The health care professional making the assessment will mentally repeat the phrase "capillary refill" immediately after releasing the nail. If color has returned by the completion of the phrase, capillary refill is considered normal (that is, the assessment is called "immediate"). If the color has not returned prior to the completion of the phrase "capillary refill," the assessment is called delayed.

Eye-Opening

Assessment of the stimulus required to induce eye-opening:

Spontaneous Response — At this point, with no further stimulation, the patient's eyes are open.

Response to Voice — If a patient's eyes are closed, his or her name should be spoken. If necessary, it should then be shouted, the important point being that any subsequent eye-opening can then be considered a response to a stimulus.

Response to Pain — If verbal stimuli are unsuccessful in eliciting eye-opening, the standard painful stimulus is applied.[1] Note: It is important to document whether the patient's eyes are closed due to swelling or facial injuries.

No Response — No eye-opening after application of above stimuli.

Best Verbal Response

Orientation — After the patient is aroused, ask the questions: "Who are you? Where are you? What year is it? What month is it?" If accurate answers are obtained, the patient is described as oriented.

Confusion — A patient who is unable to give correct answers to questions, even though capable of producing phrases, sentences, and even conversational exchanges, is termed confused.

Inappropriate Words — Notice if the patient speaks or exclaims only a word or two (often expletives). Such a response usually is obtained through physical stimulation rather than through a verbal approach, although occasionally a patient will shout obscenities or call relatives' names for no apparent reason.

Incomprehensible Sounds — An injured patient's response may consist of groans, moans, or indistinct mumbling, and may lack any intelligible words.

No Verbal Response — In some patients, prolonged and, if necessary, repeated stimulation may not produce any verbal response.

Best Motor Response

Obedience to Commands — This requires an ability to appreciate instructions. Usually these are given verbally, but sometimes they are conveyed by gestures and writing. The patient is required to perform the specific movements requested. For example, if a command is given to hold up two fingers (if physically feasible), the patient should hold up two fingers.

Purposeful Movements — If the patient does not obey commands, a painful stimulus is applied to determine whether a patient will respond purposefully to that stimulus. For example, the patient will attempt to physically repel the stimulus.

Withdrawal — If the patient does not obey commands, a painful stimulus is applied to ascertain whether the following are present: elbow flexion, rapid movement, lack of muscle stiffness, and drawing away of the arm from the trunk.

---

[1] Preferred pain stimulus is pressure applied to nail bed by pencil or other hard object.

Flexion Response — After painful stimulation, note the presence of the following: elbow flexion, slow movement, accompanying stiffness, forearm and hand held against the body, and body assuming a curled-up position.

Extension Response — After painful stimulation, note also the following: leg and arm extension, accompanying stiffness, and internal rotation of shoulder and forearm.

Face Mask

A mask which fits over the mouth and nose through which modest oxygen therapy is provided.

Mechanical Ventilator

An instrument used to provide oxygen therapy through a tube lying within the trachea (windpipe).

Serum Creatinine

A waste product from muscle activity that accumulates in the blood. It is eliminated from the blood by the kidneys. Failure of the kidneys to function properly causes the creatinine to build up in the blood. High creatinine levels are indicators of kidney dysfunction.

Hematocrit

The percent of the blood which is composed of red blood cells. The red blood cells carry oxygen; a low reading of hematocrit is usually associated with respiratory or metabolic problems.

Serum Osmolality

A measurement of the number of particles in the blood. Many of these particles are waste products. High osmolality levels cause body cells to lose fluids and become dehydrated with bad effects for various body organs.

Systolic Blood Pressure

The pressure exerted by the heart and arteries to keep the blood circulating in the blood vessels throughout the body.

Many trauma victims experience severe bleeding resulting in decreased systolic blood pressure and ultimately poor circulation of blood throughout the body.

Appendix III
CURVE FITTING

A relationship between two observed variables can often be represented by a mathematical equation.

One of the simplest relationships between two variables x and y is a straight-line equation of the form

$$y = ax + b.$$

Here a and b are numbers, sometimes called numerical coefficients, that are constant for a particular relationship, such as

$$y = 2x + 1.$$

Figure 1 illustrates this equation on a graph.

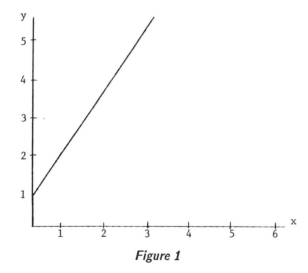

Figure 1

When a mathematical equation is used to describe a relationship between two variables x and y, the observed values frequently do not lie exactly on the line. The line is only an approximation to the observed data, which are scattered about it (see Figures 2 and 2a). The line is said to be a good fit (model) for the data if the deviations of the data points from the line are small and show no systematic pattern.

1. Does the line in Figure 2 provide a good fit to the data? _____

_____

2. Does the line in Figure 2a provide a good fit to the data? _____

_____

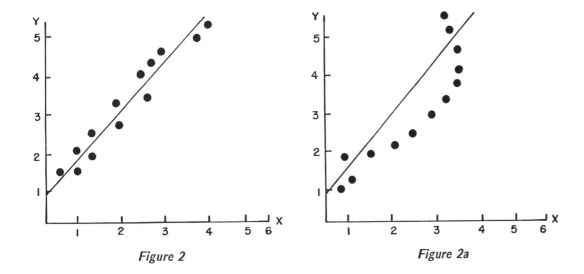

Figure 2   *Figure 2a*

The deviations in Figure 2a increase systematically, then decrease systematically, then increase systematically once again. Hence the straight line does not provide a good fit to the data. Usually it is more convenient to model such data with a suitable curve that has irregular deviations rather than a straight line that has systematic deviations. One such suitable curve is the *logistic function*. It is a popular curve for fitting probability data.

From Figure 3, Section G, page 17, you can begin to appreciate the popularity of the logistic function as a model for fitting probability data. Just as the raw data suggest, the logistic function decreases slowly at first, then steeply, then slowly once again for small values of the Trauma Score. This form is typical of many probability data sets. Note also that the deviations are small and not systematic.

Appendix IV
RESPIRATORY INDEX

The Respiratory Index, as it appears in medical journals,[2] is

$$\frac{[(P_B - P_{H_2O}\,T)F_{IO_2} - P_aCO_2] - P_aO_2}{P_aO_2},$$

where

P_B = barometric pressure (approximately 760 mmHg)

$P_{H_2O}\,T$ = alveolar water vapor pressure at the patient's
temperature (T) (approximately 47 mmHg)

F_{IO_2} = fractional concentration of O_2 in inspired gas

P_aCO_2 = arterial partial pressure of carbon dioxide

P_aO_2 = arterial partial pressure of oxygen.

Our philosophy of respiratory therapy is to keep the P_aCO_2 at 35 mmHg.
So for $P_B = 760$, $P_{H_2O}\,T = 47$, and $P_aCO_2 = 35$, the Respiratory Index
simplifies to

$$\frac{[713F_{IO_2} - 35] - P_aO_2}{P_aO_2}$$

which is the formula we used in constructing the Respiratory Index Chart.

---

[2] See, for example, M. Goldfarb, W. Sacco, et. al., Tracking Respiratory
Therapy in the Trauma Patient, *The American Journal of Surgery*, Vol. 129,
March 1975.

Appendix V
STANDARD DEVIATION

In three different classes, twenty-one students take a math test. Each class gets a different test. These are the scores and grades from each class:

Classes	F	D	C	B	A
			Grades		
1	0 0 0 0	1 1 1 2	3 4 5 6 7	8 9 9 9	10 10 10 10
2	0 0 1 1	2 2 3 3	4 4 5 6 6	7 7 8 8	9 9 10 10
3	0 2 3 3	4 4 4 4	5 5 5 5 5	6 6 6 6	7 7 8 10

1. What is the average score, $\bar{a}$, for each class? _____

   The low score? _____

   The high score? _____

The difference in the three classes can be measured in many ways. The most common measures of spread in the data are called the variance, V, or the standard deviation, S, which is the square-root of the variance. That is, $S = \sqrt{V}$.

Both are types of "distance from normal" measurements. The variance is calculated as

$$V = \frac{\sum_{i=1}^{n}(a_i - \bar{a})^2}{n - 1},$$

where a_i is the ith score, $\bar{a}$ is the average score, and n is the number of scores.

The standard deviation is

$$S = \sqrt{V} = \sqrt{\frac{\sum_{i=1}^{n}(a_i - \bar{a})^2}{n - 1}}.$$

The variance and standard deviation give virtually the same information, but in our applications, standard deviation is more useful.

2. Calculate the variance and standard deviation for each of the three classes.

Class	V	S
1	_____	_____
2	_____	_____
3	_____	_____

Special Questions and Projects

1. Write a computer program to compute P, E, and R for variables
   (a) which take on a range of values, like age or systolic blood pressure, and
   (b) which take only a small number of "values," like capillary refill.

2. Write a computer routine which can plot, with the printer, a two-dimensional graph whose "points" could be values of two indices — e.g., CHOP and Respiratory Indices, or values of $A(X)$ and the logistic function

$$P_s(A(X)) = \frac{1}{1 + e^{-A(X)}}.$$

3. The PER methodology has been explained for a single variable. However, the concept can also be applied when two or more variables are used together to make predictions. Consider the following data from 300 patients on which both systolic blood pressure and capillary refill had been collected.

	$S^3 = 20$ $D = 45$	$S = 75$ $D = 2$	$S = 21$ $D = 6$
	$S = 5$ $D = 51$	$S = 30$ $D = 35$	$S = 2$ $D = 6$
	$P < 90$	$90 \leq P < 150$	$P \geq 150$

CAPILLARY REFILL — IMMEDIATE (top row) / DELAYED (bottom row)

SYSTOLIC BLOOD PRESSURE

---

[3] S refers to the number of survivors and D to the number of nonsurvivors.

Calculate P, E, and R for these two variables when used jointly to predict patient survival.

$$P = \text{_____}$$
$$E = \text{_____}$$
$$R = \text{_____}$$

References

Champion, H. et al., Indications for Early Haemodialysis in Multiple Trauma, *The Lancet*, June 8, 1974, pp. 1125–1127.

Champion, H. et al., Trauma Score, *Critical Care Medicine*, 1981, pp. 672–676.

Goldfarb, M. et al., Tracking Respiratory Therapy in the Trauma Patient, *Amer. J. of Surgery*, March 1975, pp. 255–258.

Goldfarb, M. et al., Two Prognostic Indices for the Trauma Patient, *Comput. Biol. Med.*, 1977, pp. 21–25.

Sacco, W. et al., Trauma Indices, *Comput. Biol. Med.*, 1977, pp. 9–20.

Sacco, W. et al., Trauma Score, *Current Concepts in Trauma Care*, Spring 1981, pp. 9–11.

Answers

Answers to Exercises

1. Some possible answers: slugging average, runs-batted-in, on-base average

2. Some possible answers: competitions in diving, piano, ice skating, singing, acting, ...

3. Atmospheric pressure

4. Probable weather changes

5. A function of many variables, such as the cost of food, fuel, housing and clothing.

6. The cost of existing in today's world.

7. Body temperature

8. Possible infection

9. 11

10. 7

11. 1

12. 16

13. 2780

14. a. 1749
    b. 175

15. a. 148
    b. 133

16. 1548/1714 or 0.90

17. a. 1672/1839 or 0.91
    b. 1749/1924 or 0.91
    c. 2583/2780 or 0.93
    d. 2450/2622 or 0.93

18. 281/1714 or 0.16

19. 1400/1433 or 0.98

20. 148/281 or 0.53

24. $P = 1767/1857 = 0.95$

25. $E = 0.023(.05) + 0.35(0)$
    $+ 0.31(0.01) + 0.12(0.01)$
    $+ 0.095(0.01) + 0.069(0)$
    $+ 0.032(0.10) + 0.0038(0.05)$
    $= 0.00979$

26. $E = 0$

27. $R = .0097/2(.95) \cdot (.05) = 0.102$

28. Capillary refill

29. R

30. $P = .50$
    $E = 0$
    $R = 0$

31. **Decimal Fraction**
    Total Patients
    (1) 0.40
    (2) 0.40
    (3) 0.20

32. $P = 0.60$
    $E = 0.32$
    $R = 0.67$

33. There are many answers to this question. One such answer is given by the data:

Z Value	No. of Survivors
1	20
2	10
3	0

No. of Deaths	P_s
0	1.0
0	1.0
20	0.0

But any answer for which the P_s column contains 0's and 1's only would be correct.

34. Respiratory Expansion
$E = .115$ $R = .701$

Glasgow Coma Scale
$E = .123$ $R = .744$

Respiratory Rate
$E = .089$ $R = .684$

Systolic Blood Pressure
$E = .074$ $R = .568$

35. Best — Glasgow Coma Scale
Next — Capillary Refill
Next — Respiratory Expansion
Next — Respiratory Rate
Worst — Systolic Blood
            Pressure

37. $E = 0.1522$
$R = 0.8165$

38.

Weight	P_2
$w = 0$	0.5
$= +2$	0.88
$= +4.8$	0.99
$= -2$	0.12
$= -4.8$	0.0082

39. 12%

40. By rule 2

41. Patients 2, 3, and 4

44.

Patient	P_D
1	52
2	58
3	127
4	52
5	127
6	0

45.

Patient	C_D
1	0
2	1.30
3	3.20
4	0.50
5	7.00

46. $P_D = 10$
$C_D = 4.0$

47. Creatinine $= 1.0$
Systolic Blood Pressure $= 127.0$

48.

Patient	Points
1	20, 1
2	7, 2
3	3, 4

49.

Patient	D
1	20.025
2	7.28

50.

Patient	P_n	C_n	D_n
1	1.0	2.0	2.24
2	5.0	0	2.24
3	6.0	4	7.21
4	0	8	8.0

51.

Patient	CHOP Index
1	0
2	5.7
3	2.0
4	12.53

52. 0

53.

Day	CHOP Index
1	2.74
2	4.26
3	5.20
4	6.86
5	6.56

54. $P = 0.833$

55.

Patient	RI
1	0.08
2	1.91
3	3.02
4	above 12 or 12.385

56. $R = 0.423$

57. $R = 0.739$

58. 7

59. 8

60. 4

61. 6

62. 4.9 %

Answers to Questions
in Appendix V

1.

Class	Average Score
1	5.00
2	5.00
3	5.00

Low Score	High Score
0	10
0	10
0	10

2.

Class	V
1	16.20
2	11.00
3	4.601

S
4.025
3.316
2.145